# YOUR KNOWLEDGE HAS VALUE

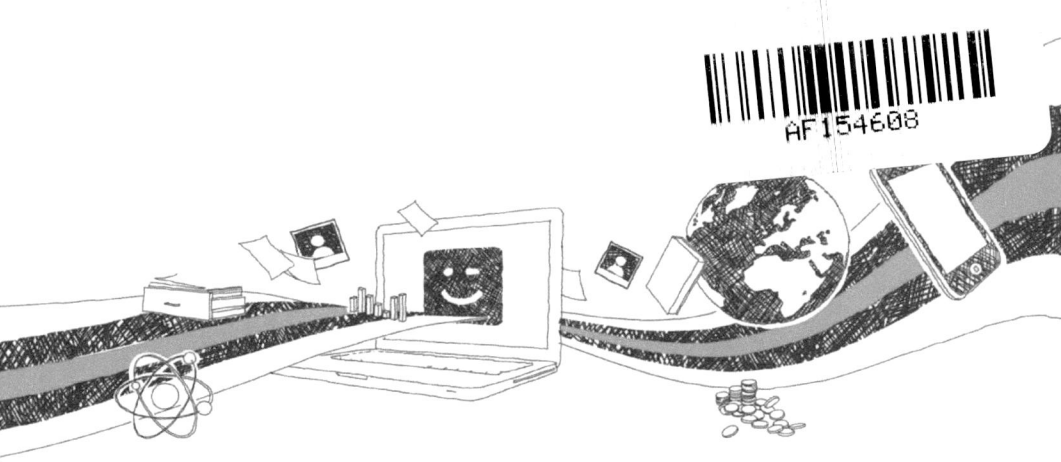

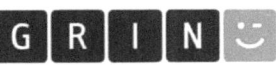

Glory Manambowoh Lueong

# Humanitarianism among Traditional Birth Attendants (TBAs). A case study of selected villages in rural Cameroon

GRIN Publishing

**Bibliographic information published by the German National Library:**

The German National Library lists this publication in the National Bibliography; detailed bibliographic data are available on the Internet at http://dnb.dnb.de .

**Imprint:**

Copyright © 2013 GRIN Verlag GmbH
Print and binding: Books on Demand GmbH, Norderstedt Germany
ISBN: 978-3-656-55615-2

**This book at GRIN:**

http://www.grin.com/en/e-book/265657/humanitarianism-among-traditional-birth-attendants-tbas-a-case-study

**GRIN - Your knowledge has value**

Since its foundation in 1998, GRIN has specialized in publishing academic texts by students, college teachers and other academics as e-book and printed book. The website www.grin.com is an ideal platform for presenting term papers, final papers, scientific essays, dissertations and specialist books.

**Visit us on the internet:**

http://www.grin.com/

http://www.facebook.com/grincom

http://www.twitter.com/grin_com

# Humanitarianism among Traditional Birth Attendants (TBAs): A case study of selected villages in rural Cameroon

*Name of Author: Glory M. Lueong*

**Author's Affiliation**: GCSC- Justus Liebig University, Giessen, Germany.

**Abstract**.

In the public health debate on how to reduce maternal deaths, Traditional Birth Attendants (TBAs) are criticised for being unable to deal with haemorrhages and obstructed labour which account for most maternal deaths. Nonetheless, in rural Cameroon, TBAs continue to practice with significantly high approval ratings of their activities by their clientele. This research used ethnographic methods to explore the following questions: what factors explain the continuous demand and supply of TBAs? Do pregnant women employing their services consider the 'risks' involved? How do TBAs themselves perceive their services to society? The findings suggested that; the prevalence of TBAs, use of their services, and clients' attitudes can be explained by a complex intertwined nexus of fear of HIV/AIDs stigma, gender, cultural beliefs and lack of access to formal health care systems. The TBAs interviewed considered their services as being humanitarian, but rural women interviewees had a more instrumental functional perception. These clients understood the risks involved, but considered TBAs to be relatively reliable safety nets when the formal health care system was seen as spatially or socially inaccessible.

**Key Words:** Traditional Birth Attendants, TBAs, humanitarianism, maternal health, formal health care system, accessibility, rural Cameroon.

## Introduction

> *My pride, fame and fortune in this calling[vocation] are not in the mansions that I have built nor in the cars in which I pull, but in the countless many who will point to my tomb and say, we are the reason for which she lived! When my tomb will be cemented, decorated and why not made a monument? That to me is true remembrance and the real value of the services that I am offering to my society (*informal discussion with Mama Tabita, Traditional Birth Attendants (TBA) from Nwa sub-Division of Cameroon, 2011)

The quote above are the words of a TBA and her take on the on the services that she offers to the society. This research explores whether or not, this is a shared view among TBAs. Also, the research seeks to understand if; there is an element of misrecognition in how the services of TBAs are perceived.

As a pre-puberty girl growing up in rural Cameroon, I was one day traumatized by a TBA who called me to assist her in a roadside obstructed labour case in Bafanji village in the North West Region(then province) of Cameroon. This call separated me from the rest of my school mates. I saw myself as a woman who will one day give birth, and the experience shocked me deeply. I could not even give the blade which the TBA asked me to give for her to use in cutting the placenta. As I struggled with my shock and fright, the bleeding woman who had been walking for kilometres to reach the nearest clinic lay helpless, while the TBA who had been called from her farm continually scolded me. This experience aroused mixed emotions in me who ended up being curious to see how a baby was born, as well as having empathy with the bleeding woman.

With these mixed feelings, I left the scene for home where I narrated the experience to my grandmother. However, unusually, she did not listen patiently that day. She instead showed anger saying that, 'they were spoiling me as a child'. She murmured for hours making very many negative exclamations as to how thoughtless the TBA had been. As though the murmuring was not enough, she left and went to inquire what had happened. To her shock, she met other women busy trying to curb the woman's bleeding which did not stop until she passed away. She came back weeping as she narrated the story.

In 1996, just three years after the first scare, we as a group of secondary school girls coming back from school were called to stand around another woman giving birth on the roadside in Nchimekone quarter Pinyin, Santa Sub-Division so that, our male mates should not see how the baby was being born. I felt sorry for both the baby and mom, but then wondered what really was wrong with women. However, I grew older; I continued to encounter similar birthing situations and came to realized that, it is a common phenomenon in most parts of rural Cameroon.

In this regards, the present research sought to understand the dynamics of maternal health service provision in rural Cameroon where women are caught between employing the services of TBAs and using health centre/ hospital facilities(here after, 'formal health care system'). To do this, the rest of this paper is structured as follows. The following part presents the research problem and questions, part three describes the research methodology, part four presents the major research findings, as well as their policy implications for rural maternal and reproductive health service provision. Throughout this research, the term 'skilled attendants' (qualified nurses and midwives) will be used to refer to professionals in the 'formal health care system'. The use of 'skilled' in this way has nothing to do with implying that TBAs are unskilled. It is simply for differentiation purposes since both TBAs and midwives have skills.

## Problem of study

Prior to the introduction of Western medical practices, women gave birth at home and each society had a way to identify, follow up pregnancy and subsequently attend to delivery through TBAs[1]. Statistics published in 2004 for rural Cameroon, report that 57.5% of the women who die from a birthing related circumstance die in the house[2]. Similar statistics in other parts of the developing world have raised a global call for concern about women's health especially that, 99.6% women who die in childbirth live in places where access the formal health care system is difficult[3] and 60% of the births occur outside the formal health care system, assisted only by TBAs, family members, or without any assistance at all[4]. In this situation therefore, TBAs who cannot handle haemorrhage, sepsis, eclampsia, obstructed labour and complications of abortions which account for 50 to 75% of these deaths[5] are criticised for a significant part of high maternal mortality.

View these; mainstream policy has been to train TBAs in biomedicine which is said to be capable of handling haemorrhage, sepsis, eclampsia, obstructed labour and complications of abortions thereby reducing the high rates of maternal mortality[3, 6]. This has since the 1987 Safe Motherhood Initiative, sparked wide scale research to understand the contribution of training TBAs in the battle to reduce maternal mortality. However, the researches came to quite divergent recommendations. For some, training TBAs can help reduce maternal mortality[7, 8]. For others, the training of TBAs is not productive and sponsors should consider alternative health investments[9]. Nonetheless, some of the researchers still argue that, although governments are being persuaded to ban TBAs[10,] they are not to blame[11] because, majority of the deaths are not defined by the TBAs[12].

Following these mixed stances taken by the various researchers in their policy recommendations, policy, at least at the level of implementation, is also mixed when it concerns TBAs in rural Cameroon. In some instances, they are trained[7] while in others; they are not trained and have remained the scapegoats blamed for high maternal mortality thereby, making the subject of TBAs and their services an issue of controversy in rural Cameroon. But overall, despite "the actions taken by the government and some of its development partners to reduce maternal mortality[23]" there has been no significant reduction in maternal deaths in the country since 1990[21]. Rather, according to the available health statistics for Cameroon, a woman dies almost every hour from complications related to pregnancy and childbirth[22] with mortality rates that range between 669 deaths per100.000 deliveries[23] and 705 deaths per 100.000 deliveries[24]. To this effect, the subject of TBAs and their services remain an issue of controversy in rural Cameroon.

Considering this death rate and the tendency to blame it on TBAs[2], the present research sought to understand the following: which factors account for the persistent demand and supply of the services of TBAs even in rural areas where there is a formal health care system? Do pregnant women employing their services consider the risks involved? How do TBAs themselves perceive of the services that they are offering to society?

According to Pereza and Tih, the ideal scenario, is when "every woman would give birth in a health facility in the presence of a professional health worker[25]". However, considering the socio-cultural and economic contexts of most developing countries, maternal health needs to be tackled as a public-health issue whereby there is a consideration of community interventions as being complementary to care received in health facilities[25]". On the same footing, Kamga and others in a 2012 study on *"the appreciation of Traditional Birth Attendants' services in Cameroon in the context of HIV/AIDS in Cameroon[26]"* show that, out of a total of number of 2566 survey participants, 74.6 % of them living in rural areas showed a satisfactory appreciation of the activities of TBAs.

Connecting this high appreciation of TBAs in rural Cameroon, it could be thought TBAs could play a very important and complementary role in the public health endeavour of reducing maternal mortality in rural Cameroon. Moreover, this qualitative rating of the activities of TBAs in rural Cameroon, rhymes very well with quantitative national statistics which suggest that, of a total number of 4547 rural inhabitants sampled, up to55.6% of them received maternal assistance outside a formal health care system," 18.6 % of whom were assisted during delivery by a TBA , 29.7 % assisted by a relative or other and 7.3 % delivering on their own[27]". View these, it undeniable that TBAs play a significant role in rural maternal and reproductive health provision. However, what remains unclear is why, rural women continue to highly appreciate their services whereas, most if not all of them cannot handle haemorrhage, sepsis, eclampsia, obstructed labour and complications of abortions which account for majority of maternal deaths [5]. To this end, it is important to understand the factors that account for the persistent demand and supply of the services of TBAs. Also, it is important to understand if pregnant women employing their services consider that there risks involved? And finally, how TBAs themselves perceive of the services that they are offering to society and what motivates this perception? This are the questions that the present research sought to answer.

## Methodology

This paper is part of a larger ongoing research on "community responses to maternal deaths: perceptions, causes and interventions". The findings analysed here in, were collected during a three months research in Cameroon between the months of October to December 2011 using ethnographic methods.

Cameroon is located in the gulf of Guinea and shares boundaries with Nigeria to the west, Chad to the north, Central African Republic to the east, Gabon, Equatorial Guinea and Congo to the south. The country has an estimated population of about 20 million inhabitants[33] with 48% living in urban areas and 52% living in rural areas[26]. In total, 51% of the Cameroonian population are women among whom there is a birth rate of 33births/1000 population, 56% of which occur in rural areas[34]. The research sites can be seen located on the Country's Map in Figure 1.

*Figure 1: Map of Cameroon with an indication of the research sites*

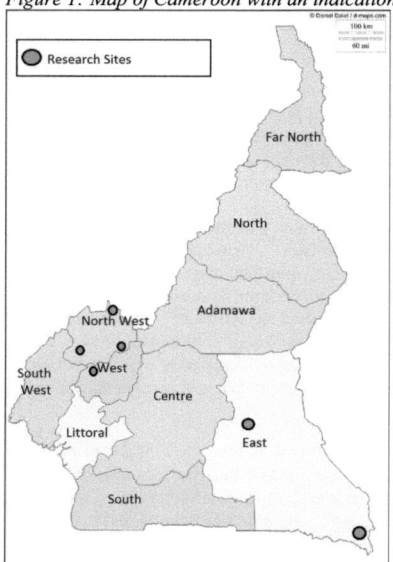

*Source: Copied but adapted from 'Daniel Dalet/D-maps.com' by the Author.*

As can be seen from Figure 1, this research took place in three (Northwest, West and East) of Cameroon's ten administrative regions. In the Northwest, the research was conducted in Mezam, Ngohketunjia and Menchum Divisions. In Mezam Division, Mbelluh (including Mudum and Njimbat) in Bali sub-Division, Fingue in Tubah subdivision and Pinyin in Santa subdivision were visited. In Ngohketunjia Divion, the research took place in Bafanji and Bamumkumbit in Balikumbat subdivision. In Menchum Division, Benakuma, Bosung, Benader all in the Menchum Valley subdivision were visited. In the West Region, the villages of Memfung and Bagam in Galim subdivision of Bamboutus Division were visited. In the East Region, Banana in Moloundu of the *Boumba et Ngoko* Division and Myos, Lossou, and Koumanjab of the Upper Nyong Division were visited.

The choice of these three Regions was based on the following: the East Region is reported to be one of the regions in the country where more deliveries are attended to by TBAs because of poverty and long distances to access health facilities[26, 2]. The Northwest and West Regions are reported to have relatively fewer women who employ the services of TBAs[26]. In this light, conducting the research in these regions was perceived to be the best way to find out what is central in the practice of TBA beyond the already well known factors of poverty and lack of access to the formal health care system.

The choice of villages within these regions was determined by differential access to formal health care. Mbelluh, Pinyin and Bafanji fitted into the criteria of choice, and were also villages in which firsthand personal experiences of births outside the formal health care system were encountered in my past.

The research was conducted with TBAs, skilled attendants in both the private and confessional sectors, rural as well as 'indigenous' women. The women participants were aged between 23 and 50 years and included the following categories:

- 'indigenous' (Mborroros and Baka 'pygmies'),

- women who were expecting their first babies and had never attended prenatal care, but hoped to rely on the assistance of a TBA to initiate them into the birth process,

- women who never used the services of a skilled attendant for all their births,

- women who started giving birth in the formal health care system but later switched to TBAs,

- women who started to give birth with TBAs but switched to skilled attendants,

- women who switched between TBAs and skilled attendants depending on the necessities (if complicated as indicated by cultural norms, the services of a TBA were sought but if a normal and simple pregnancy, it did not matter), and

- women who had family relationships with TBAs

In total,

- 20 in-depth Interviews were conducted with women from all the categories described above.

Five Focus Group Discussions lasting between 90 to 120 minutes were also conducted with;

- women who started giving birth in the formal health care system but later switched to TBAs,

- women who started to give birth with TBAs but switched to skilled medical assistants ,

- Women who switched between TBAs and skilled nurses depending on the style of the child.

Four 'Participant Observations' were undertaken with TBAs (three in the homes of a TBAs and one in the home of a pregnant woman). Six informal group discussions lasting between 45 an 90 minutes were conducted with indigenous women (Mborroro and Baka). Seven key informant interviews lasting between 60 and 90 minutes were conducted with skilled attendants in both the private and confessional sectors. Five life history interviews were conducted with TBAs and women who gave birth to all their babies using the services of a TBA. After an interpretive analysis of the data, it was observed that, several factors accounted for the persistence of TBA practitioners in rural Cameroon which will be discussed in the following parts of this paper.

# Findings

The research found that, poor access to health facilities, cost of services, behaviour towards clients, belief systems, gender norms, social pressure and the fear of HIV/AIDS stigma all worked to support the demand and supply of TBAs who in turn perceived their services as being humanitarian to a society in need. This finding explains why, although TBAs were aware that they could become the scapegoats blamed for high maternal deaths, they continued to offer their services which on the most part were free. To systematically present the research findings, eight factors have been identified.

### 1. System of health care provision
Health care in Cameroon can be obtained from a wide range of providers spanning from the government, private, mission hospital/health centres, local patent drug stores, pharmacies to traditional or folk medicine practitioners[13]. In conventional care, government providers are cheaper than the private and mission/confessional providers. However, in the countryside, mostly private and mission providers are present and even when a government provider exists; they end up being extremely understaffed. This is because; the nursing profession in Cameroon is a female-dominated profession[13]. So, most often, skilled attendants posted to rural areas end up abandoning their duty posts to join their spouses in the urban areas especially if, there is no political influential elite from the region whom the nurses feared that s/he could cause their salaries to be blocked. In this frame of mind, most skilled posted to rural areas would not forego urban facilities for the mud, dust, hills and poor social facilities of those people in the 'bush' as they call it.

On the part of the skilled attendants, they complained about not having good schools for their children, not being able to get access to some other social facilities as well as what they termed their extremely 'small salaries' which they sometimes ended up spending more than a tenth of it just to go and cash it from banks which are located only in urban areas. In rural settings, government employed skilled attendants who managed to stay at their duty posts tended to do what they wanted, how they wanted and when they wanted, thereby, leaving the people at the mercy of either the private or mission providers which when available were expensive, or to traditional providers whom the populations consulted both as their primary providers of health care[13] as well as for psychosocial[14] problems. At this juncture, pregnant women were confronted with wishfully wanting to seek a skilled delivery assistant and feasibly resorting to TBAs.

### 2. Confrontations: women forgoing their farming days to access modern health facilities versus exhausting schedules on the part of skilled attendants.

In this section, I discuss how constraints surrounding access to the formal health care system and significant sacrifices made by rural women to access the facilities confront with the exhausting and stressful schedules of skilled attendants who have cater for people coming from very many villages. Such circumstances resulted in dysfunctionalities whereby nurses blamed their clients (rural women) while women on their part blamed nurses. In comparison, TBAs can be seen as being humanitarian in the sense of presenting a caring human face.

> "...Villages without roads and without health centers still exist...
> It takes days to move from one of these villages (Tinta) to the nearest hospital (Akwaya)
> [in Cameroon].Please, I wish to invite WHO and other advocates of the abolition of

*traditional birth attendants to live in one of these villages and have one baby there. In August 2006, I visited a village and was told that I was the first health authority to come there. These people are voiceless, powerless, and poor. Who will speak for them[7]*.

This quote from the head of one of the confessional health provider in Cameroon gives a hint about the health service accessibility situation in most villages in rural Cameroon. The country faces a "shortage of qualified health personnel with 16 nurses and midwives per 10,000 inhabitants; 2 physicians per 10,000 population and <1 pharmacist per 10, 000[26, 29]". In other regions of the country, one very sparsely equipped hospital serves 14 villages (approx.6000people)[33].

In the Menchum Valley sub-division, one of the sites where this research took place, there is only one district hospital for 19villages (very distant apart with poor transport facilities such that, women estimated that, it took them between 5 to 8 hours to trek from their villages to the district hospital). Visits to some villages in the sub-division revealed the details shown in Table 1.

**Table 1:** Availability of modern medical facilities to some of the researched villages

| Name of Village | Situation |
|-----------------|-----------|
| Bosung | No health centre |
| Benader | One Baptist health post with one nurse |
| Benakuma | The district hospital |
| Benahundu | No health centre |
| Benebenge | No health centre |
| Vikroo | No health centre |
| Beter | No health Centre |

*Source: Composed by Anyenju in March 2011 during missionary activities in the subdivision.*

Despite this absence of modern medical facilities however, most women did not immediately choose to employ the services of TBAs. On the contrary, most of them reported travelling to the neighbouring villages and sometimes semi-urban areas to receive skilled assistance. As barriers to seeking skilled professional assistance, women mentioned distance, transport facilities and the lack of understanding by nurses as being challenges that made them to resort to the TBAs as will now be discussed.

In Mbelluh-Mudum and Njimbat, the nearest health unit was 8kms away with no motorable road from the village to the health unit. Occasionally, four-wheel drives vehicles forced their way through, but no such public transport existed for the inhabitants of this village. Women in these villages as well as in others in Menchum valley had to trek distances between 8 and 15kms to access maternal health services. In other regions *"only 40% of women can access government health services. [Thus,] most women deliver at home with TBAs [since] it can be difficult to reach the hospitals due to bad roads, transport costs and the long distance to travel, which is up to 28kms for some women[33]"*. In villages where 'public' transport was available, pregnant women had to experience travelling in overloaded vehicles with as many as eight passengers in a standard four passenger car, a situation that was extremely stressful and even risky for the life of the women and their unborn babies.

More so, travelling to other villages/semi-urban centres to access modern medical facilities meant that these women had to forgo two or more farming days each time they went for clinic /consultations. This was because, by the time that they finished with their clinic lessons and individual consultations, the return car which often made only one trip per day (especially during the rainy season) was already gone. Thus, the women had to spend the nights with their friends and/or relations to board a return car the next day. In cases when these women managed to comeback the same day, they complained about being overly tired for work the next day because of the shaking in the vehicles which did not often have shock absorbers on potholed roads. This loss of farming days was very significant to the productivity and incomes of these women, especially when they had to miss a market day which only came up once in a week.

To this end, most of the women interviewed preferred to skip clinic than to miss their market days or eve (when they normally go to harvest what to sell on the market day). This choice to skip clinic in a bid to meet up with their financial needs revealed to be a source of problem between them and the skilled attendants the next time that they travelled to the clinics. According to these women, the nurses who 'insulted', shouted and sometimes refused to attend to them did not understand the dynamics and difficulties of live in their villages. As another participant aptly put it:

> *The baby will come to add to the number of mouths that I have to feed. Also, I have to look for what to pay hospital bills, buy her napkins and omo with. so, I can not only be following what the nurse said and forget to work hard because, when the child will cry of hunger or will be sick, I will have to spend money which if I do not work for now, then that time when I am home [because I just gave birth], who will give to me?* (In-depth interview with a pregnant woman in Memfung, Dec.2011)

On the part of the skilled attendants interviewed, they pointed out that, village women were very negligent about their health and were putting them (the skilled attendants) in difficult professional situations. To these attendants, village women ought to think properly before conceiving, so as to give their babies the best of care required. Some of the interviewees, who had switched from skilled attendants to TBAs, identified this problem of distance, obstruction of their farm days as well as the subsequent misunderstanding by skilled attendants when they skipped clinic as being the principal causes of their switch to TBAs who understood their situations. This misunderstanding between the women and skilled attendants is what I have coined confrontations of access to modern medical facilities versus exhausting schedules of skilled attendants.

Added to this lack of understanding was the fact that prenatal and postnatal lectures were given to women in groups. In this process, women came and took reception numbers until 10 or 11am (depending on the clinic and the region). After this time, the skilled attendants gave lectures to the group followed by individual consultations based on the reception numbers. In this way, women who trekked from distant villages came to the clinics late, took last reception numbers and were consulted last when the skilled attendants were tired, working overtime or under other constraints. At this point therefore, both the clients and skilled attendant felt frustrated against each other whereas, it was not the making of either of them. It is simply put it, the result of the confrontation of two structural dysfunctionalities rather than the will of either of the parties.

Thus, women facing this situation and counting the cost (physically, socially, economically, and culturally) resorted to switching to TBAs for subsequent births while trying to justify their despair by making statements like: *"even in the clinics and hospital, women still die. Death at birth is an issue of luck" (Aginess during an in-depth interview in Mbelluh, 2011).* Nonetheless, the point here is not to quickly recommend that, bringing health centres closer to rural women will stop them from employing TBAs. While spatial access to the formal health care system played a role in determining the demand and supply of TBAs, the cost of these modern health services, gender, culture and belief systems, language, the social location of TBAs as well as the fear of HIV/AIDS stigma revealed to be other factors which influenced the dynamics of the demand and supply of TBAs.

## 3. Financial and social cost of using the formal health care system.

As already mentioned above, public health care providers are cheaper than mission and private providers who in some cases were the only providers in rural areas. In both cases, the natures of provider-client relationships as well as the cost of services were determining factors for women seeking skilled birth attendants. When women chose to receive medical attention from the private/confessional providers where they could pay later, they had to sacrifice their 'last dime' as well as mingle with women from higher social classes which were not always easy:

> *"I gave birth to my first child in the hospital and my box was a very old one. Even my bed sheets and everything I used to dress the bed. I felt too ashamed when I saw how other women's beds were. It was as though I am the last person in this world. So, I decided that if my husband cannot buy new things. I will not go there again. I will call a TBA to deliver me here in the house where only I and my family will know how we live our lives" (Rose, in-depth interview in Bafanji, 2011)*

Considering that, TBA assisted birth did not require a display of riches or status[1], women who used them felt more comfortable. In the same light, TBA's believed that, they were serving humanity with gifts which only they inherited. Like Mama Franscica, a TBA aptly illustrated:

> *"God cannot take his time to build a child and put in a woman's womb and give you the talent to remove it and you leave her to die because she does not have money! I count it joy and will never hesitate to offer my service whenever I see a case in need. You cannot understand how many children that I have delivered and today the village is full of kids. When you yourself look at their bright faces in school uniforms, tell me, aren't your happy? Then, what more of me who takes part in their birthing process? Even on plantain leaves, the baby's first cry sparks immeasurable joy and gives colour to my life!" (In-depth interview in Bafanji, 2011)*

This situation described by Mama Francisca very much fits well with the needs of poorer women with unproblematic pregnancies who needed someone to help them deliver. This reflects a very different situation compared to government providers which appeared to operate on the principle of "money before service or remain neglected even if it means death[16, 17]" .The documentary in the references provides an image of some of the daily realities of women in rural Cameroon, where due to structural challenges, a provider of public health has tended to confuse the distinction between emergency and money[16] *la distinction de l'urgence de l'argent* as the French would put it. In an opening question to me, my interviewee Mary asked:

> *Tell me what you will do, if you struggle and travel this long distance, leaving your children in the house without any senior just to go to clinic and they [the Nurses] do not even look at you as though you are feeling the same pains that they too feel when giving birth. They instead start insulting you and asking for huge sums of money whereas your mother-in-law is there delivering other women for free and nothing is happening to them" (In-depth Interview with Mary in Mbelluh, 2011).*

In this case, it was not a question of paucity of formal health care system services, but that of cold reception and lack of warmth which forced rural women, especially those of the underprivileged social classes to resort to TBAs especially as, their services were rendered free of formal charge[15]. But, just as it is difficult to convince humanitarian organisation about the dangers of their aid activities among beneficiary populations, so too, it is challenging to criticise the health risks in the services which TBAs are offering. A more humanitarian environment is an important aspect of the practice which health policy makers need to reconsider. It is not enough to frame TBAs as being unskilled without seeking to understand why their services are valued. Flagging the lack of skills of TBAs misses the point that, the TBAs and their clients perceive them as humanitarian with valuable indigenous knowledge.

In this way, what would have been a complementary[21] partnership in rural maternal health provision has become one of strife where each party is quick to point to the faults and incapacities of the other thereby; leaving the population underserved while each party (TBAs and modern health services) justifies its authenticity and know- how.

This is the case that Dorothy evokes when, she says *"Traditional Birth Attendant is derogatory term"* and

> *My grandmother was one of these so called "birth attendants," yet, she could do anything when it came to the birthing process. This includes the delivery of a breech, twins, any complication during birth. How many skilled midwives or specialists today can do this type of complicated birth without technology? Are these skilled attendants really skilled? And where are the skilled attendants when the so-called traditional birth attendants provide the majority of primary maternity care in many developing countries[31]*

Whereas, providers of modern medical facilities on their own part give sharp and blunt warnings to rural populations, arguing that, "going to a traditional birth attendant for childbirth is an act of risking [the] death of a mother or a newborn or both as these fellows are not knowledgeable and thus in case of any complication deaths occur[28]". TBAs do not see "their lack of training as a problem but, rather point to the non-cooperative and disrespectful attitudes of providers in hospital settings as the most important issue affecting their work. [Adding that,] the continued demand for their services [is due] to its high quality and wide-ranging nature as well as to their sensitivity to their clientele's needs, which contrasts with the abusive treatment many women receive in hospital settings[18]".Another TBA, conversant with the maternal health delivery system in Cameroon went further to ask what proofs that they the TBAs) are the causes of maternal deaths when "in Cameroon, [the] notification of maternal deaths is not mandatory and maternal death audits are not institutionalized[21]".

To this end, it is important for policy makers to take into consideration the above analysed confrontations which arise from structural dysfunctionalities thereby leading to harsh behaviours, neglect and indifference thus, creating a space for finger pointing.

### 4. Language and communication between women and health care providers

The research found that, in some cases, women from indigenous and marginal communities especially the Baka faced language difficulties when they tried to explain certain things to skilled attendants for example that, some medically recommended practices and nutritional habits were not permitted for pregnant women in their cultures. This difficulty, they said made the skilled attendants to construct them as being stubborn. In the same light, a lack of understanding about how the modern medical facilities functions made some of these women to go to clinics and not take reception numbers whereas, on the most parts they were the earliest. Thus, the skilled attendants tended not attend to them during individual consultation since it is based on reception numbers. With this lack of understanding, these women rather complained of being neglected by medical personnel who to them were 'discriminating' because they consulted other none 'indigenous' women first whereas they (the 'indigenous' women came much earlier). Adama, a mborroro woman further added during an interview that:

> *"Those 'doctas'[referring to skilled attendants] are too wicket! I can never go there again. When you go there, no matter how early you go, they will only treat you last and will even be insulting you. It is only that when I was sick, the 'docta'[a trained medical doctor] said I should come to the hospital to give birth but I can never go there again. They treat you as though you are not a person" (In-depth interview with Adama, Bamumkumbit, 2011)*

In this light, the women tended to resorted to TBAs who understood their language, were more clients friendly and were always available when solicited. In extremes, these women delivered on their own without any assistance as has been reported by another study in rural Cameroon, where "Madame Pelagie delivered all her babies by herself with no problems [and when] asked if she felt frightened during the births, she replied no and that, she was more frightened of going to the hospital, she cut the first baby's cord with a bamboo knife, the others with a razor blade[33]". Such women who delivered on their own without any assistance are estimated to make up 7%[27] of the total births in the country. Belief systems were also another factor that played a determining role in the demand and supply of TBAs in rural Cameroon.

### 5. Pregnancy and child birth belief systems

> *"Another reason given for not attending a health centre or hospital for delivery was the cultural tradition of giving birth to your first born child in the house where you were born. Encouraging women to attend hospitals and health centres appeared to be the biggest challenge for health workers[33]".*

Human reproduction from an anthropological perspective is a cultural event that is dependent on social relationships and cultural meanings[6]. Thus, pregnancy and child birth have a whole lot of beliefs[14] and practices surrounding them with each ethnic group having a set of beliefs that justify their very existence as a group[19]. In most parts of rural Cameroon, there is reference to the TBAs as being the ones who best master these belief systems and can educate the younger women especially on dietary prohibitions during pregnancy.

Among the Baka for example, Table 2 shows prohibitions and taboos .

**Table 2:** Taboos relating to pregnancy and child birth among the Baka in East Cameroon

| Prohibition | Concerned individuals | Possible consequences |
|---|---|---|
| Urinating in a stream | Pregnant women | Miscarriage |
| Having sex with a man other than one's husband | Pregnant women | Complications during delivery |
| Having sex while breast feeding | Nursing mothers | Illness and possible death of the child |
| Killing an animal | A man whose wife is pregnant | Death of the fœtus and miscarriage |
| Tying an animal | A man whose wife is pregnant | The child suffers from malformations or is tied by its umbilical cord at birth |
| Splitting the head of an animal | Pregnant woman | The child is born with a cleft palate |
| Eating the brain of an animal | Pregnant women | The child will have a snotty nose |

*Source: Gathered by Author during own research but first published by Plan Cameroon[32]*

In other villages, some of the beliefs observed were that, obstructed labour is due to witchcraft whereby a jealous relation or friend has tied the baby in the womb. Also, there were beliefs which associated haemorrhage to totemism. In this belief, it was said that, if a woman is totemic and gets pregnant as a human without dissociating herself from her animal in the forest, the animal will also get pregnant, and if by some chance, the animal delivers before the woman, she is doomed to die during birth and this inescapable death would be signalled by continuous bleeding after birth (haemorrhage).

Most skilled attendants in rural areas were insensitive to these beliefs because, as already analysed above, in some subdivisions, one clinic/ hospital served more than 10 different villages thus, women who came from far off villages had norms and beliefs which nurses were not familiar with. Thus, the nurses were not knowledgeable about the beliefs and were thus, not able to sensitize the women about the medically incorrect beliefs/myths.

Moreover, due to the nature of clinic classes and individual consultations, there were hardly Question and Answer (Q&A) sessions between skilled attendants and women on issues of cultural norms and beliefs about pregnancy and birth. On the contrary, in some cases, medical practices such as, hindering the presence of family members during delivery[19] significantly angered women from some villages who held to beliefs about the presence of an elderly woman during birth such as to counter mystical forces that could attack the woman or the unborn baby.

More costly about this absence of understanding of beliefs was the fact that, in most of the villages, there was a belief which associated difficult delivery to infidelity of either of the couple during the pregnancy. So, when a woman started to get a difficult delivery, the remedy as stipulated by the traditional belief was that her husband should not give any money or whatever to the woman until the baby was delivered and all after birth bleeding had ceased. Otherwise, the baby and mother will die.

Such beliefs which associated obstructed labour to the infidelity of either of the couple, and in turn demanded that, a husband should neglect his wife so as to save her life, ended up yielding very deadly consequences for poor women who employed modern medical facilities. These women who at the same time were struggling with the pain of obstructed labour as well as the torture of an assumed infidelity were left all alone. No one to console them as their husbands who could have saved the situation either financially or morally were kept out of the scene and the nurses due to a lack of understanding, failed to give the much needed moral and psychological boosting as they had no idea about the cultural battle going on in the women's minds.

In such situations, the services of TBAs were very much solicited, not so much because they could better handle obstructed labours but because, they could give the psychological support needed both by the women and their in-laws. Sometimes even, the TBAs went as far as suggesting rituals that could counteract the situation. At this point, the TBAs did not see themselves as experts who knew more than skilled birth attendants. Instead, they saw themselves as people 'called and talented' to the service of humanity. TBAs in this case were thus a network of mutual aid and psychological support between the women and their families[19].

This situation further indicates that, there is need for modern health care providers to properly integrate into the broader social and cultural contexts of the rural world which they seek to serve. This may be done by simply censoring the myths and believes about pregnancy and birth within the vast regions that each hospital/clinic serves and plan educative sessions during clinic lectures. In this way, skilled attendants and their clients will trade on almost the same level of understanding when it comes to beliefs, myths and what is medically correct about pregnancy and birth. Another factor closely linked to this belief system which significantly played a role in the negotiation for access to maternal health care was social pressures from within the family social structure.

### 6. Social pressures from within the family social structure.

In rural Cameroon, depending on which culture one is dealing with, in-laws play a very crucial role in the stability of a nuclear family. In the domain of child bearing, the situation was even more complex because most husbands believed that, their mothers and sisters are wells of experiences on which their wives need to draw. This reduced the decision making margin of the women who at the same time had to respect their in-laws so as to keep their marriages. Mama Ngwi, a mother-in-law for example recounted how the fear and stubbornness of her daughter- in-law made them to lose a child and she was ready to look for another wife for her son if Emilia (her daughter-in-law) continued to be stubborn because, she (Emilia) was married and brought to increase the family by giving birth.

Mama Ngwi recounted that, a witch had been tying the baby in Emilia's womb for a longer period than normal (10months), but when she (Mama Ngwi), told her (Emilia) to go with her to consult a TBA who was at the same time a traditional doctor and was best placed to solve their problem, she (Emilia) refused and said that, the doctor said her baby is cross bridge and she needs to be under medical supervision until she gives birth. While still narrating the story, Mama Ngwi with a strong expression of bitterness asked me that:

> did she (Emilia) think that she was the first woman to give birth? Whom did she want to tell who about birth? Yes, they went and wasted money, but the baby still passed away. Now that she is again pregnant, she has learnt and does not argue

*anything that I tell her again. We do not refuse the hospital but it has its own things*
*that it can cure she said* (In-depth interview, Menfung, Dec.2011)

From this narration, and others that came up during the field work of this research, it can be read that, social pressure from within the extended family structure play a significant role on women's decisions in the domain of making the choice of a birth attendant. Women's choices were moderated to ensure they would keep their marriages. This situation is closely related to the next factor which is that of gender in procreation.

## 7. Gender in procreation

Family planning helps couples to stay within their desired family size while still enjoying the pleasure of marriage. However, for most women in rural Cameroon, the decision to adopt any family planning method threatens the stability of their homes. In this part of the world, gender based violence against women is not only limited to the physical, cultural, systemic and institutional. It also extends to the psychological level where it keeps women under constant subjectivity thereby, hindering them from actively determining the size of their families.

In most cases, the participants reported that, they had no voice in deciding how many children they wanted to have and those who even tried to, said that, it was very risky to the stability of their marriages. Those who were monogamously married said that they risked having their husbands marrying second wives to have more kids while, those who were already in polygamous marriages said *"he will love your mate who has more kids or is still giving birth"*. In most rural families, the nuclear family size ranged from 8 to 10 irrespective of their incomes. This size was either aimed at providing labour on the farm, resulted because of the search for a particular sex (often males) or the search for love from husbands in polygamous homes.

On the contrary, the skilled attendants interviewed were very unaware about these phenomena and rather tended to sensitize women about family planning lessons. In some cases[2], skilled attendants cautioned that, women should stop having children. When this happened, the women tended to shy away from clinics and continue to give birth using the assistance of TBAs than lose their marriages or have a co-mate come in like Marthe related.

> *'My husband said he wants 10 children. When I had the 6th child, I had a problem and the nurse asked me to stop. When I came and told him, he said that, it is my plan with the nurse but that, it is ok he will marry another woman. So, I had to get pregnant again. When I went to register for clinic, the nurse was very angry and shouted at me. Since then, I have had these other two in the house with my mother in-law'* (A case that came up during a Focus Group in Memfung, West Region.2011)

In this way, a separation of the nursing profession from the gender question turns to produce a skew in favour of the demand for TBAs who willingly supply their services because of their proper understanding of the existing gender question. Thus, women only resorted to TBAs not that there was a strong preference for homebirths[5, 30]. Another factor closely linked to this which also played a role in negotiating for access to maternal health care was the fear of knowing their HIV/AIDS status as well as being stigmatized with it.

## 8. The fear of knowing their HIV/AIDS status and being stigmatized.

In the Cameroonian formal health care system, there exist HIV/AIDS tests for women who register for prenatal programs. Nonetheless, although the literature[7] suggest that HIV/AIDS sensitization campaigns have gone a long way to persuade women especially mothers to know their status, field findings suggested that HIV/AIDS related stigma scared most women(especially those in a vulnerable marital position) away from wanting to know their status. Pauline illustrated this when she said:

> *Can one really escape from this 'thing outside' [HIV/AIDS]? My co mate has many boyfriends and our husband too is not free. 'Wuush' I cannot dare to go to the clinic with this pregnancy? The moment they tell me that I am HIV positive, I will die. Knowing that you have it kills faster than not knowing. I will stay like this and give birth in the house. After all, death is death (In-depth Interview with Pauline in Memfung, West Region, 2011)*

Most women depending on their conjugal context tended to be very scared of knowing their HIV/AIDS status and thus resorted to TBAs who did not test for the disease.

## Conclusion

This paper argues that, the general model of maternal and reproductive health which is being used for policy implementation seem to miss out the whole phenomena of "the rural" which has been overly supplanted with the concept of poverty. There is a rural dynamism which cannot be ignored. A rural woman may even have the money to consult a medical facility but, like in the case of Pauline who is married in a polygamous home and lives in a community where it is known that, when you are told not to breast feed your baby, it means that you have HIV/AIDS, she for fear of the unknown will resort to use the services of a TBA who is there just to help get her baby delivered. A midwife in one of the villages, made an allusion to the same when he said that:

> *Working is this village is very difficult. The stigma attached with having HIV/AIDS makes it very difficult to even tell a pregnant woman her status because you just do not know the next step she may take. Some have stopped attending clinic and others even, I only see them when the disease starts manifesting on their children. (In-depth interview with a midwife, October 2011)*

Summarily, it can be said that a nexus of intertwined factors contribute in explaining how rural women negotiated for access to maternal health care. However, it is important to highlight that, there were some factors that were common to all three regions while others were to a large extend region specific.

On the one hand, factors that were common to all regions included: the humanitarianism of TBAs who were readily available to offer their services and 'expertise', cultural beliefs and taboos related to pregnancy and birth, fear of being exposed to the stigma of HIV/AIDS, gender in procreation, transport difficulties and lack of access to modern medical facilities.

On the other hand, factors that were more specific to the Northwest region were harsh behaviours of skilled public nurses and gender(family size and family planning: where women shied away from skilled attendants because they were advised to stop giving birth or use birth controls). In the West Region, factors of gender (polygamy: giving birth to more children such as to be loved by husband and in-laws irrespective of whether it is home or in the hospital) were more dominant. The factor of language was predominantly common among the Mbororo and 'Pygmy' who felt suppressed/not understood when they tried to express themselves. From these, an attempted framework has been put forward to explain the humanitarianism of TBAs.

Thus, there is a complex mix of socio-economic, cultural and political challenges which are widespread in rural Cameroon and understood by TBAs. These challenges operate in an intertwined complex nexus called 'the rural'. But women from 'the rural' with its challenges need maternal and reproductive health services which formal health care system is meant to provide. Thus, the TBAs and formal health care system are obliged to interact in the framework illustrated in Figure 2.

Figure 2: A frame work for understanding the Humaniterianism of TBAs in the context of rural maternal and reproductive heath

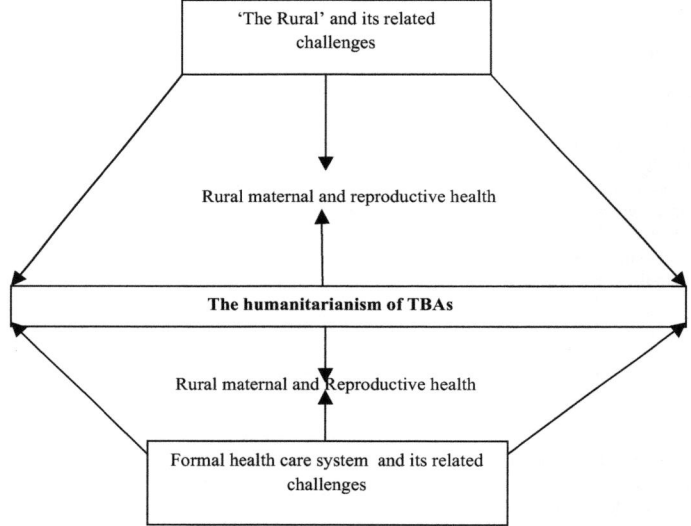

In Figure 2, "The rural" and it challenges consist of factors like: lack of access to modern medical facilities, bad roads and transport system, fear of being stigmatised versus rural resilience strategies in an era of HIV/AIDS, gender and cultural norms, lack of education, poverty, the pressure to maintain a conjugal stability.

The humanitarianism of TBAs is captured in the perception that they consider their services as services to humanity and do not withhold it where needed especially that, it fits very well into the social solidarity that exist in rural areas. By nature, TBAs are warm, friendly, and receptive. Predominantly, their services are readily available, accessible, and cheap and in most cases free, they are masters of traditional belief systems. They also hardly talk to women about their family sizes and rarely do HIV/AIDS tests (except those who have been trained). So, fearful women remain ignorant of their status thus, free from stigma. Also, the nature of their service delivery erases the visibility of class difference among clients. Per their social positions, they are often parents, in-laws, friends or relations so can also potentially exert significant influence on route choice.

The modern medical system challenges include: limited infrastructures, understaffing, extremely stressful work schedules, poor or no equipments, financial limitations and poor management.

This research suggests that, the factors nurturing the perceived humanitarianism of TBAs in rural Cameroon are more complex and intricately linked to the phenomenon of 'the rural' than do public health literature and political talks suggest. Rural women are well informed about the possible risks and dangers in being delivered by TBAs. However, this phenomenon of 'the rural' which is a complex and intricately linked network of gender, culture and belief systems, poor transport, poverty, fear of stigma, lack of education, language and resilience strategies tend to confront with challenges faced by modern health care systems to oblige women to resort to using the same services which they would dread if a second choice were offered to them.

The paper argues that, rural people have different resilience strategies to cope with changing incidences of global epidemics. To some extent, resorting to TBAs is resilience to the strong stigmatisation of HIV/AIDs which public health policy has not yet adequately tackled. Therefore, while training some TBAs to test for HIV/AIDS [7] has been well applauded for curbing the incidence of mother to child transmission, tackling the stigma which forces some women to resort to employ the services of TBAs is more important for rural maternal and reproductive health in general. The fact that women continue to seek the services of TBAs, even when the formal health care system is available, does not mean women are unaware of health risks. Thus, policy 'experts' may reconsider decrying the work of TBAs and blaming maternal deaths primarily on the lack of medical facilities and delays caused by poor transport infrastructure contributed to the high incidence of maternal deaths[20].

## Contribution of Authors

This research was conceived and designed by the above mentioned author of this work (Glory M.Lueong). She also collected and analysed the data.
Thomas Mike Anyi Nju a aided the data collection by providing the tabularised situation of availability of health centres in the Menchum valley of North west region of Cameroon (Table 1) above. The Author of this manuscript approves of the manuscript and Thomas Mike who aided in the data collection also gave his consent for the publication of the information the Table 1 above.

## References

1.      Petitet PH. L'art des matrones revisité. Naissances contemporaine en question Faustroll, Descartes 2011.
2.      NIS. Troisième Enquête Démographique et de Santé, 2004; Available from: http://nada.stat.cm/index.php/catalog/23/overview. Retrieved on 05.07.2012
3       Petitet PH. Les matrones et la reduction de la mortalite maternelle, une contribution au debat. Global Health Promotion. 2011 December 1, 2011; 18(4):31-4.
4       World Health Organization. Coverage of Maternity Care. A Listing of Available Information. World Health Organization, Geneva. WHO/RHT/MSM/96.28.;1997.
5       Walraven G, Weeks A. Editorial: The role of (traditional) birth attendants with midwifery skills in the reduction of maternal mortality. Tropical Medicine & International Health. 1999;4(8):527-9.
6       Hay MC. Dying mothers: Maternal mortality in rural Indonesia. Medical Anthropology. 1999;18(3):243-79.

7       Wanyu B, Diom E, Mitchell P, Tih PM, Meyer DJ. Birth Attendants Trained in "Prevention of Mother-to-Child HIV Transmission" Provide Care in Rural Cameroon, Africa. The Journal of Midwifery & Women's Health. 2007;52(4):334-41.

8       Jokhio AH, Winter HR, Cheng KK. An Intervention Involving Traditional Birth Attendants and Perinatal and Maternal Mortality in Pakistan. New England Journal of Medicine. 2005; 352(20):2091-9.

9       Smith J, Coleman N, Fortney J, Johnson J, Blumhagen D, Grey T. The impact of traditional birth attendant training on delivery complications in Ghana Health Policy Plan 2000;15:326-31.

10      Rasch V. Maternal Death and the Millennium Development Goals. Danish Medical Bulletin, 2007; 54:167-9.

11      Goodburn E, Chowdhury M, Gazi R, Marshall T, Graham W. Training traditional birth attendants in clean delivery does not prevent postpartum infection. Health Policy Plan 2000; 15:394-9

12      Wollast E, Renard F,Vandenbussche P, Buekens P. Detecting maternal morbidity and mortality by traditional birth attendants in Burkina Faso. Health Policy Plan.1993;8(2):161-8.

13      Fongwa MN. International Health Care Perspectives: The Cameroon Example. Journal of Transcultural Nursing. 2002;13(4):325-30.

14      Tsala-tsala J. Ethnopsychologie des interdits pendant la grossesse. Cahiers Sociol Econom Cult Ethnopsychol. 1996; 25:86-8.

15      Fru AE. The role  of Traditional Birth Attendants (TBAs) in  maternal delivery   in the Mbatu community,NW province Cameroon:  University of Yaoundé I; 2008.

16      Kristof ND. Save our Mothers: A video about prudence's death in Cameroon In: Nathaniel N, ed. *Save Our Mothers*. USA: New York Times, 2006.

17      Agendia A. Cameroon's free fall health system: Two videos shock the world. In: Agendia, ed. *Participating in Positive Change* 2010.

18      Izugbara C, Ezeh A, Fotso J-C. The persistence and challenges of homebirths: perspectives of traditional birth attendants in urban Kenya. Health Policy and Planning. 2009 January 1, 2009;24(1):36-45.

19      Beninguisse G, Brouwere VD. Tradition and Modernity in Cameroon: The Confrontation between Social Demand and Biomedical Logics of Health Services African Journal of Reproductive Health 2004; 8(3 ):(152-75).

20      IRIN. Malawi: President lifts ban on traditional birth assistants. Guardian Development Net Work 2010.

21      Hounton S.  State of the world's midwifery.2011. Available online at http://www.unfpa.org/sowmy/resources/docs/country_info/short_summary/Cameroon_SoW MyShortSummary.PDF. Retrieved on the 09.11.12

22      Mbouzeko R. UNICEF: 'Roadmap for care' aims to improve maternal and newborn survival in Cameroon. 2009 . Available from: http://www.unicef.org/infobycountry/cameroon_49572.html. Retrieved on the 10/11/2012. Retrieved on 08.11.12

23      Ndi NE. Increased maternal mortality in Cameroon blamed on poor family planning, allvoices. 2010. Available online at www.allvoices.com. Retrieved on the 06.11.12

24      Hogan MC,  Foreman KJ,  Naghavi M, Stephanie, Ahn SY, Wang M, Susanna M M. Maternal mortality for 181 countries, 1980–2008: a systematic analysis of progress towards Millennium Development Goal 5, Institute for Health Metrics and Evaluation. 2010.

25      Pereza F, Muffih TP. The Use of Midwives and Traditional Birth Attendants in HIV Care, Volume 3: Developing Pathways and Partnerships, In: Marlink RG, Teitelman ST, eds. From the Ground Up: Building Comprehensive HIV/AIDS Care Programs in Resource-Limited Settings. Washington, DC: Elizabeth Glaser Paediatric AIDS Foundation; 2009. http://ftguonline.org. Available online at http://ftguonline.org/ftgu-232/index.php/ftgu/article/view/2046/4089. Retrieved on the 12.11.2012. 2004

26      Kamga HLF, Njimoh DL, Nsagha DS, Assob NJC, Nde Fon P, Njunda AL, community survey of appreciation of Traditional Birth Attendants' services in Cameroon in the context of HIV/AIDS. Scholarly Journal of Medicine. 2012;2(6):84-88.

27      Cameroon 2004: Results from the Demographic and Health Survey. Studies in Family Planning 2006; 37(1):61-65

28      Saiboko A. Tanzania: Traditional Birth Attendants Incompetent. allAfrica.com. 26 July 2012.

29      Médard, JF. Décentralisation du système de santé publique et ressources humaines au Cameroun», Le bulletin de l'APAD, n° 21, Un système de santé en mutation : le cas du Cameroun. 2009. http://apad.revues.org/document35.html. Retrieved on 7. 11. 2012.

30      Fowler GM, Shaffer N, Tih PM, Greenberg AE, Karita E, Coovadia H, and De Cock K M, Role of traditional birth attendants in preventing perinatal transmission of HIV Marc Bulterys, medical epidemiologist, BMJ. 2002; 324(7331): 222–225.

31      Dorothy. Traditional Birth Attendant is derogatory term, Alliance of African Midwifes, 2012 .Available from: http://www.african-midwives.com/2011/traditional-birth-attendant-is-derogatory-term/ . Retrieved on the 13.11.12

32      Plan Cameroon, Culture and Traditions of the Baka Pygmies, done for Plan Cameroon by Rased, 2006.

33      Askamum, Life as a mother in Cameroon: A UK midwife blogs her visit with UNICEF, midwife Nicki Westoby's diary of her time in Cameroon. Available online at: http://www.askamum.co.uk/News/Search-Results/Current-news/Pampers-Diary/ .Retrieved on the 7th.11.2012
34      WHO: Cameroon country statistics. Available online at www.who.int/maternal_child_adolescent/countries/cae.pdf .Retrieved on the 13.11.2012

---

[1] On the most part, when women give birth in rural clinics, they have to carry their suitcases to theclinic where they spend between three to seven days depending on when: the baby's navel is healed, when they have money to pay the hospital bills and or when the baby is circumcised. This has

often been a display of riches as women show off with having bought a new set of napkins for every child, using expensive baby products like Babe chlorante etc. This intimidates poorer women who feel unfit for the environment.

[2] Especially where they judged that, a next conception will expose the women to deadly risks.